GW01313412

# DEMENTIA AND NELLIE DEAN

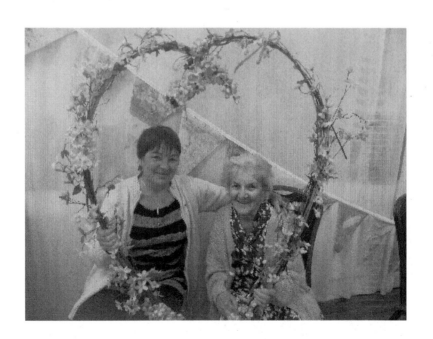

# Foreword

Nellie Dean – My very own Guardian Angel!

My mum became my best friend too. She had always been a good and loving mother, but became an even more special best friend when dementia struck.

We had 11 years of laughter and fun together because of dementia. Through the bad times, there were many good times.

Every person experiences dementia in their own way. The story of Nellie Dean explains how my mother endured.

These days, I hold her close in my heart.

Thinking: "I should phone".

Is she still here with me?

I like to think so!

---o0o---

# Introduction

Mum, Elsie, was one of nine children and she had already seen dementia take several of her sisters. She was the only one left. I watched dementia take her too and cannot say that, at any time, we "Lived well". We learnt and we managed. Through education and understanding we lived "better". The disease was devastating for mum but also for our whole family. I am the third of her four children. Many people write their stories leaving a message for the future. I simply want everyone to know how brave my mother was and mention some of the things that I learnt on the way.

Dementia is a term which refers to physical diseases of the brain. For the types referred to in this book and many other rarer forms - **there is no cure**. It affects mainly the elderly but can also affect younger people too. Sometimes there is a family link but not always.

# Chapter 1

## *ELSIE aka NELLIE DEAN*

I am Jane Moore from the UK and, for 11 years, I looked after my mother who was diagnosed, in 2006, with Alzheimer's disease and Vascular Dementia.

A rollercoaster of sadness and happiness, of personal triumphs and new horizons. I still see her peeling potatoes, making pastry, gardening, washing up and picking fruit with me.

I see her in the local public house singing her favourite song "Nellie Dean".

I hear people fondly calling her Nellie Dean in town. Singing in the car and dancing at the café – wonderful memories I will cherish forever.

It was a privilege to deeply be with mum and get to know her, more than I ever would have, had it not been for dementia.

We laughed and sang, walked and played together every day!

Then there were the bad times when nothing was right for her, angry and crying, looking for her home and following me wherever I went all day long. (Now mum is gone I would give anything for her to be following me again!)

I thank my husband for being so patient with us both!

"Shadowing" is the term used in dementia for a person who needs to stay close and it's a behaviour that is difficult to change.

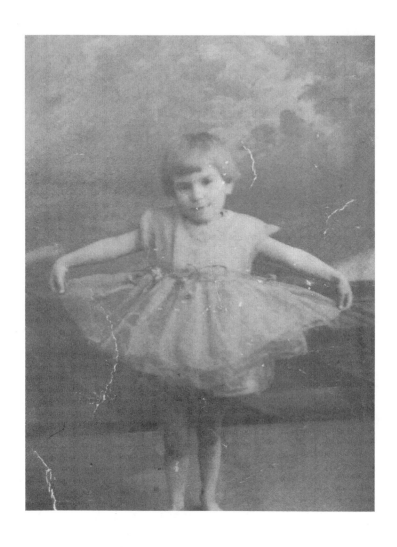

My mother, Elsie, was born 1921 in Neasden, in London, in a road overlooked by the power station.

The houses along her road were all Railway cottages. She was one of 9 children living in cramped conditions. Money for food and treats was in short supply. However, love was in abundance. My grandfather worked as builder/maintenance man for the railway houses along the road. He said that if he had a threepenny bit in his pocket, he was a rich man! At weekends mum worked alongside her sister Nell in the workers' canteen and bosses restaurant at the Power Station. It was here that she learnt to cook basic and fancy foods. There was no money for Elsie to attend a Convent for schooling but she was determined to go there. During the war years she worked at the General Electric Company. After the war, she married her childhood sweetheart, my father, who lived in the same road and they were convinced that life was going to be good. They eagerly awaited the arrival of their first born - but

David John had severe Spina-bifida and only lived for 2 hours.

To say they were devastated is an understatement. My parents went on to have three more children, 2 girls and a boy. I recall mum making wonderful petit four cakes for school events and other fairs and holding dinner parties for friends. Mum and dad often dressed up and went out to dinner-dances.

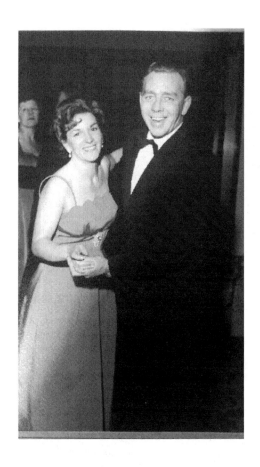

Then, when I was 12, my family moved to Norway where my father started the first steel mill, in Bergen. We all enjoyed skiing, skating, boating on the fjords and other sports, and it was a wonderful grounding for life.

5 years later we returned from Norway and settled in Surrey, where we rebuilt an old house and rescued a couple of horses. Mum loved to dance and the Strauss Waltzes were her favourite. She was also fond of cooking and gardening but above all, she loved to paint.

She was a staunch member of Tadworth Art Group and some of her work sold at local exhibitions.

She also liked to read and collected a huge selection of books – particularly on art.

## Now let me introduce you to My Nellie Dean!

For years my mother looked after me, cared for me and loved me. Then it was my turn as she became more forgetful and her life became confused. At the time, I was living in Cornwall and, whenever I visited her in Surrey, the neighbours would say that she needed to be cared for. They knew her well and it became apparent that she was becoming confused, leaving the front door open at night, going out leaving the cooker on and spending a huge amount of money on charities, among other things. So in 2005, Mum eventually agreed to move in, with my husband and I, in Cornwall and I gradually became her memory, her thinker and her full time care partner.

Some of the unusual behaviour, I describe in this book, arrived with the onset of mum's dementia.

So whenever my mother became angry, repetitive, or even more overjoyed than she usually was, I called her Nellie Dean! The pet-name began when I discovered the song "Nellie Dean" was her favourite. She was still the same person who raised me up as a child and loved me - despite my *own* tantrums, at times, growing up too! My father had passed away some years before and mum had continued to live on her own and enjoy her art groups, many friends and social activities. She would walk for miles across the heath, where she and dad loved to be, and was happy.

When she moved in with us, mum would sing her favourite song wherever we went and I soon learnt the words.

When she sang in the pub one afternoon, and other shops in Camelford, she became known locally as Nellie Dean!

The lovely publican, Jo, had placed a huge bottle on the bar with mum's picture on the front to fundraise for Alzheimer's Research. "Elsie – our Special Friend" it said! A gentleman at the bar said he would put a fiver in the jar if mum sang for him! And, of course, she did! Her favourite version was by Florrie Ford:

"THERE'S AN OLD MILL BY THE STREAM, NELLIE DEAN

WHERE WE USED TO SIT AND DREAM, NELLIE DEAN"

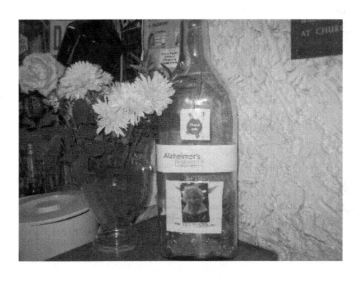

After a couple of years mum had a scan and was formally diagnosed. We were in the garden when a car arrived in the yard and a well-dressed chap in a suit approached us. He said he was my mother's consultant from the hospital and had come to show us the scan results. He said he had phoned to arrange his visit and spoken to mum. Well, it seemed to me as though he had a great deal to learn about dementia!

July **2009** Note written by Mum:

*Thursday 30th "to see doctor. Test results? Yes! Alzimer's! For what it's worth knowing?! PTO Have Alzhimer's find out how to spell it!"* (I noticed mum's spelling was leaving her! She was once told she was eligible to join Mensa and her English language was always excellent)

Mum had many friends gathered through a very social lifetime and, sadly, all but 2 real friends ignored her once they knew she had dementia. I am eternally grateful the friend who continued to write to mum, despite never receiving a reply. It seems stigma still exists around diseases that people don't understand. My "friends" too drifted away one by one and mum, my husband and I all felt prisoners to the disease.

Sadly, it often happens that friends don't understand and only a few remain in contact.

Chapter 2

## *PURPLE ANGEL*

In 2010, I sought companionship, support and learning, on facebook, on a site called Dementia Aware. The site had been set up by a dementia sufferer Norman McNamara – who prefers being called just "Norrm" by his friends. Diagnosed at just 50 years, Norrm was determined to raise awareness of dementia in his town of Torquay in Devon, where he lived with his partner Elaine. To date there are over 21,000 worldwide members of Dementia Aware, exchanging information and supporting each other. Norrm was struggling to receive any understanding in his local shops so decided to dedicate the rest of his life to raising awareness and to let people know of his own experiences. Norrm, at first diagnosed with Alzheimers Disease, was eventually diagnosed with Lewy Body type dementia. This type of dementia gives rise to hallucinations and a loss of life skills - very debilitating and frightening.

Norrm designed "The Guide to Understanding Dementia" poster. He asked on the Dementia Aware Facebook page for someone to make him a logo to award shops and businesses. He had asked staff to read the poster and learn a little about the symptoms of the disease. I doodled an angel – "my angel" is what Norrm calls Elaine, his partner and carer - and coloured it purple (the colour for health). Norrm was delighted. Thus the Purple Angel Campaign was born. People from all over the world wanted to join in, raising awareness, in their local towns and cities, and became ambassadors for the campaign. Many of these people were carers and people with memory loss too. Some were working in the field of dementia care, charity or fundraising.

The campaign spread, much to our surprise, and within 5 years the Purple Angel was being used in over 50 countries around the world with nearly 1000 ambassadors and growing by the day!

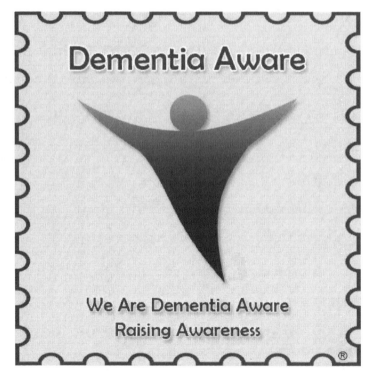

Now I continue to watch and monitor in amazement. One small purple angel spearheading some wonderful projects throughout the world.

My eternal thanks go to our Purple Angel Ambassadors for all their hard work.

Our Purple Angel ambassadors are responsible for new Memory Cafes; Radio Shows and even projects in countries where there is little support or recognition of dementia at all. Books; blogs; hospital training; shops and business awareness, befriending, Day Care, Ponies, MP3 players and the list goes on.

Now the Purple Angel can be seen in many towns in the UK, and abroad, letting people know how they can support people with dementia and make a difference to people's lives.

Norrm, Elaine and myself have continued to raise awareness and have now opened and run memory cafes in both our towns.

Memory Cafés are great places to relax and just be yourself!

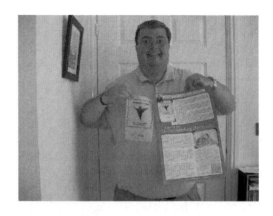

Norrms with the Guide to Understanding Dementia poster and the angel sticker.

In the beginning Norrms said to me: "You don't know what you are getting into!"

As time went by, I think he and Elaine realised that they too had no idea, at that time, in more ways than one what the future held!

We are now the firmest of friends.

Lewy Body Dementia is caused by protein deposits in the brain. Symptoms can vary but include loss of life skills; hallucinations; tremor; lack of spacial awareness; speech problems and unsteadiness. Thinking; memory and movement can all be affected and Parkinson's like symptoms can develop.

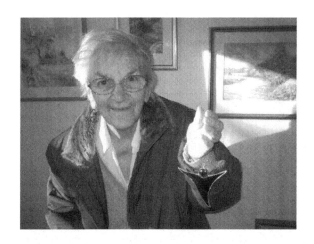

THE INTERVIEW: It was 2011. Mum and I began our quest to make our local town of Camelford dementia aware. We were interviewed for the local news on TV. Mum, by this time, was living in the local care home, but agreed to give an interview about dementia. She was very proud of the Purple Angel that her daughter had made for her. "I had that Alzheimer's once" She said to the interviewer. "You can cure dementia by drawing!" and, *yes*, she was almost right! Drawing gave her the enjoyment and absorption she craved and she could forget all her worries.

Just like favourite music, drawing can gladden the soul and keep the brain active.

A positive outlook can change the outcome of a disease such as cancer so why not for dementia?? Mum mentioned drawing because it was all consuming and enjoyable and when she could no longer draw or paint her pictures, repeated renditions of "My Nellie Dean" took her to that same place of solace and joy.

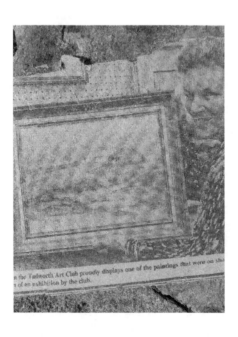

THE FAVOURITE SONG:

There's an old mill by the stream, Nellie Dean

Where we used to sit and dream, Nellie Dean

And the waters as they flow. Seem to murmur sweet and low

You're my heart's desire. I love you.
Nellie Dean                    By Henry W Armstrong 1905


Music! We all need music in our lives. That special place for each of us when we listen to our favourite tunes.  Relaxing, revitalising, it awakens the soul, brings back memories and makes you feel alive inside. I discovered that music can also do even more.


Music is one of the only activities that stimulates and uses the entire brain. It can also help with pain and stress and stop dementia in its tracks for a short while.

## Chapter 3

## *CAMELFORD*

To begin our dementia aware community, we needed to raise some funds for printing. Mum and I grew plants together and then sold them in the High Street!

We sang Nellie Dean and ate Fish and Chips on the pavement which mum would never have done in the past!

We made enough money to cover printing of the poster and to pay for some purple angel stickers. It was also an excellent way to provide space at home to grow more plants together!

We had many great days outside in the garden, keeping busy and feeling useful.

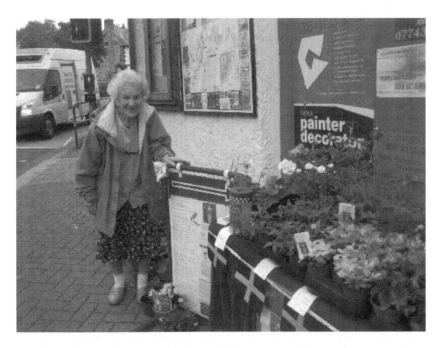

Our plant sale in aid of the Lewy Body Society.

We continued to visit local shops but it was clear that Nellie Dean could not help me with this anymore! She insisted on telling all the shopkeepers that she had Alzheimer's once and now was cured!

Of course, even today, many years after, we still have no cure for these dreadful diseases.

So I continued alone, as it began to upset her to talk about it.

Since then, I have visited over 700 shops and businesses, in 4 towns, and given talks about dementia to numerous groups and clubs.

I return to those shops every year to update new staff and spread a little more awareness.

From year to year, these shopkeepers remember my visits and I am often asked questions about dementia from staff and customers alike.

Each year, there are many new shops that have opened up and, as we live in a holiday area, there is quite a high turnover of temporary staff each year.

Not being able to recognise having a mental illness is called Anosognosia which causes some people to reject any diagnosis. It is a real condition and, in dementia, may come and go.

# Chapter 4

## *DEMONS*

I needed some time to support my husband, when his mother passed on, and the funeral was many miles away. Due to her failing health, Nellie Dean could not attend and would not agree to respite care.

A nightmare scenario ensued when a friend offered to take care of Nellie Dean for a night. My Nellie Dean was not having any of it!

*My diary: 7th to 11th Nov. 08 My mother in law's funeral. My good friend B here to take mum to hospital for her appointment.*

The evening before, we were all to go to a charity evening, making sweet-bags to raise funds. Mum began to cry because her fingers hurt making the bags up. I told her "best stop doing it then". She said she didn't like my attitude, and the way I talk to her, and that she was going to live with my sister in Surrey.

Meanwhile, mum told me she didn't think my friend B was a good friend for me. I responded that I was surely allowed to have whoever I wanted as a friend. She said she would get an ambulance to the scan at the hospital so I told her it was all arranged and not to use a valuable ambulance space. I trust B with my house, my money and my mother. Unfortunately, B caught a cold so I had to ask a neighbour to be on standby for the hospital, so I could go to the funeral which was many miles away in Norfolk. Nellie Dean told me not to talk to her and go away. Refusing lunch and still in a mood on Friday, Nellie Dean had an argument with B, then went across the road to the neighbour's house.

I suddenly remembered seeing a pan on mums stove in the annex and it was about to take fire with smoke everywhere. I fetched her home.

I told Nellie Dean she was too angry to come out to the charity evening so she decided she would get a taxi, or that the neighbour would take her. The neighbour was out.

I told Nellie Dean that she had nearly burnt the house down. She said it wasn't much and that she'd done it before in her old home. She was annoyed that I had fetched her back from the neighbour, so she phoned my sister and asked her to come and pick her up the following day and find her a house to rent.

I rang my sister and explained how mum was behaving and that she was not able to live in a rented house on her own and *who* was going to look after her? My sister was beginning to see there were more serious problems than she knew about and what could she do?

Later Mum cried saying that she was sorry about everything and was happy in Cornwall.

On the Sunday I left for the funeral in Norfolk and B took over. B took Mum out for lunch and then to Tintagel. Nellie Dean kept on to B about the troubles and told her she didn't want to drive with her. Eventually, the neighbour was asked to drive mum to the scan.

My friend B was tormented by Nellie Dean, even when she tried, later, to go to her room for some peace.

The kind neighbour eventually took mum to the hospital for the scan and all of us ended up distressed and very annoyed.

The demons had taken over. I had needed to support my husband and I knew this was not the way Mum would have wanted for me to live my life.

## Chapter 5

## *OUTINGS TOGETHER and KINDNESS*

Walking was always fun, especially in the countryside. One day we did a 3 mile walk through some woods! Mum had always been a good walker and was, physically, very fit.

We went everywhere together. Car Boot sales, carnivals, garden visits and so on.

Once, upon returning from a carer's afternoon at the Eden Project, where we had enjoyed an interactive singalong, we both felt relaxed and happy. The lunch had been provided and I had watched a cascade of chopped egg fall from the roll Nellie Dean was eating, surrounding us both in a sea of egg and crumbs! For a change, I was happy to let someone else do the clearing up!!

We sang, we laughed and we danced.

As we drove back home, Nellie Dean started to sing. "Land of Hope and Glory" – It was great to see her so happy!

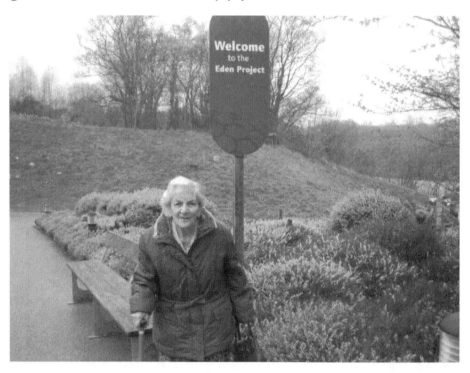

## THE CONVENT AND "ELSIE'S SECRET"

We would sing in the car together, the pub and the high street, and many of the shopkeepers joined in her song!

Little did anyone know that Mum was gleefully immersed in her own little secret, for the song "Nellie Dean" was sung to her by the boys of her teenage! I am grateful my mother did not elaborate, but it was obviously one of the best times in her life!!

She met my father when she was 14 years and fell in love with him. She was a very determined lady and managed to earn her scholarship to The Convent of Jesus and Mary in London. She was so proud of her achievement.

Her joyful attitude to life proved a challenge for most of the nuns who, I am sure, would have wished her to behave in a more refined way! Nellie Dean recalled to me the fun of playing truant in the park!

However, the kindness of the nuns left a lasting impression on Mum. They taught her well. She was christened Church of England and eventually confirmed at the Convent.

My mother married in blue to her sweetheart (her one and only love) and the colour blue remained her favourite till the end of her days along with the brightness of yellow.

Yellow is thought by some to be the last colour to be recognised in dementia.

Through joining the Convent face-book page, we realised that Nellie Dean was the oldest living pupil.  I was messaged by one of the old girls, saying that mum was invited to a re-union in London.  Unfortunately Nellie Dean was no longer able to travel any distance. The younger pupil messaged that, if we could send some pictures and information, she would make a presentation which would be shown at the reunion.

How lovely! A prayer was also said for Nellie Dean which I know she would have appreciated, if only she had known.

I am sure mum would have been thrilled to know how much it meant to everyone to see the life story of their most elderly pupil.

.

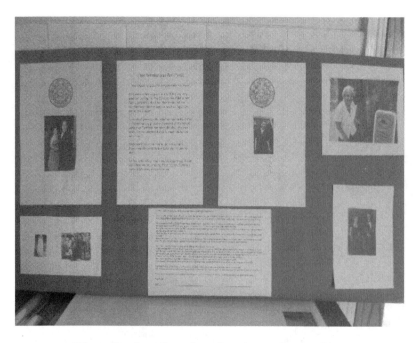

*The display for the Convent Re-union.*

Mum had always found great comfort from being involved with the church and had great respect for the congregation, although she much preferred to make the tea for everyone!

A Christingle service we went to was a bit slow for Nellie Dean. She had been given an orange, a candle and some sweets but, when I looked, there were no sweets left!

They had been eaten, one by one, throughout the service and we were left with just the orange and the candle!

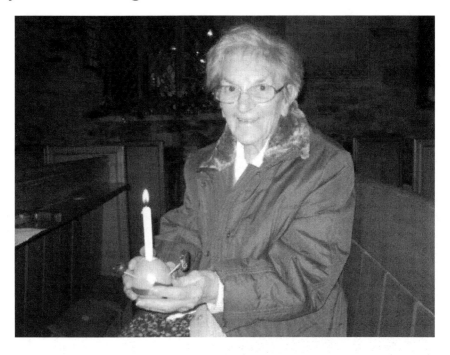

Later we were to join the dementia friendly church services which were set up as part of the dementia friendly community with Launceston Memory Café. Mum could no longer attend our local church when her hearing and memory failed her.

Concentration was also problematic, so the smaller, shorter service made her feel accepted once again. She immediately felt as though she were among friends. Mum even sang "Nellie Dean" and "All Things Bright & Beautiful" during the service and everyone clapped!!

One day, at the dementia friendly church service, she surprised me! She was a nurse in the war – or so she told the vicar! I kept quiet having learnt that it is not good to argue with a person who has dementia! The vicar was very tactful and told Nellie Dean it was a wonderful vocation!

There was the time Nellie Dean met Maggie Thatcher! (!!!)    The vicar just replied again: "How wonderful!"  Then Nellie Dean became a WREN in the war. (REALLY?!!)

It must be wonderful to be anything you like!

It was at this time that my granddaughter Amy, then age 7, wrote a story for Nellie Dean. A beautiful story called "The Little Purple Angel". Here is an excerpt:

ONE DAY THERE WAS A LITTLE PURPLE ANGEL. HER NAME WAS ELSIE.

SHE LIVED IN A BIG MANOR HOUSE WITH BEAUTIFUL FLOWERS EVERYWHERE.

ONE AFTERNOON ELSIE WAS PLAYING WITH HER TEDDY. SHE THREW IT SO HIGH IT WENT IN THE BUSHES. SHE CRIED "OH, NO – I MUST GO AND GET IT". SO SHE WENT INTO THE BUSHES AND THERE WAS A SPARKLING PURPLE PATH. SHE FOLLOWED THE PATH AND SHE SAW A PRINCESS PURPLE ANGEL.

By

AMY LLOYD-HUGHES

Some of the happiest times were spent with Nellie Dean sketching in the park together or simply walking and looking for squirrels. Things that are free are the joys of life and it's the small things in life that so many people don't value.

Take care to join the person where they are and even if you know there are things said or done which you don't think are real – they are certainly real in the mind of a person with dementia. Don't leave them by themselves with these thoughts but join them, empathise, say: "Tell me about it".

## Chapter 6

## *THE SOCIAL BUTTERFLY*

My mother had several jobs when she left the Convent, but never stayed in any one for long. At one of the places of work, her boss called her a butterfly because she was flitting from job to job and never stuck at anything!!

However, she stuck at the Memory Cafes. We were also members of our own Café in Camelford, where we met a Professor from the USA visiting. She was on a fact-finding mission looking into English memory cafes to see how they were set up and run. She would go back to the USA to start the very first café there and we understand there are now hundreds more that have sprung up across the United States.

Other countries have since set up Purple Angel Memory Cafes and I keep in touch and see their success on Facebook.

They all vary, but most have a common theme of activities, music and lots of cake!

We are trying to introduce fruit to our café but the cake remains the most popular!!

At the cafes Mum would find a new partner to dance with and loved to take part in everything that was going on. She became known to many as "The Dancing Lady".

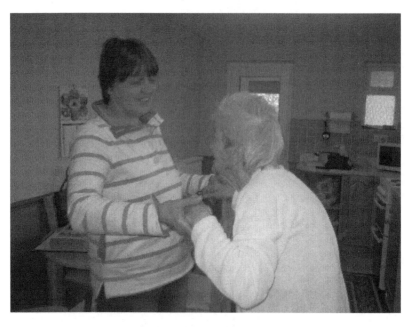

*Sister Sal dancing with mum.*

Keeping social has been shown to be beneficial to delaying the progression of dementia.

Just before the onset of Alzheimer's and Vascular Dementia, it was mum's 80th birthday. We celebrated, danced and ate in a big hall filled with many good friends of hers. It was an evening to remember! This was about a couple of years before she could no longer manage to live on her own and moved to Cornwall.

In all the 11 years Nellie Dean had dementia she was able to deny it and professed to all that there was nothing wrong. However, I knew full well that hiding it was for my benefit and the only way mum could carry on.

Her 85th birthday arrived. We held another party and some good friends of mine kindly played music for her and sang. I realised how much life had changed for my mother in those short years since her 80th party.

It really was the "school of hard knocks".

By the time her 90th birthday came around, there were no friends at all. The only way I could make anything better was to learn as much as I could and I enrolled in several courses on the internet for dementia and learnt about the brain. I was discovering new ways to communicate with Nellie Dean which was my salvation and hers!

Alzheimer's Disease is the most common dementia type. Symptoms vary from person to person depending on which area of the brain has been affected. Proteins build in the brain to form plaques and tangles which lead to the loss of nerve cell connections and eventually to the death of cells and shrinkage of brain tissue.

Chapter 7

## *CONFUSION*

One morning, 9.30 in the kitchen, I made tea and toast with banana for breakfast. I had made a bad choice, as she said her mouth was sore. I suggested a walk in the local park but mum said she didn't feel up to it. I went out and bought some Mouthwash instead.

During the morning mum said: *"When are you taking me to a home?"* I said "We are not going anywhere until art class this afternoon".

Then she asked why we weren't going to see the old people – she meant the cognitive stimulation class on Mondays which she usually enjoyed. I said: "They are not old! Some of them are 20 years younger than you!" I let her know that today was not the day for her class, by which time she had forgotten all about her question on the care home.

Lunchtime arrived and I made scrambled egg and we went to art class. Art had meant a great deal all her life, always sketching and drawing wherever we went. Mum felt dizzy and said she should not have come. She said her gums were sore, so I gave her a small paracetamol and said I would take her home.

A few minutes later she felt better and wanted to stay at the class, then suddenly felt unwell and tearful again.

I said I would take her home so we packed up and went. She was angry with me on the way home, saying that I didn't think much of her – she would have stayed resting at the art class. I said I could not paint with her not feeling well.

She said she would go back to live with my sister, Sal, in Surrey. We arrived home and I told her to rest. She came back at me angry and tearful, 5 times, saying she would have stayed at art and that I had made a mistake. (I should not have *told* her to rest – I should have *asked* instead). I went to fetch our neighbour as mum always talked to him ok. When I returned she was sorry – said it must be dementia. Thank goodness – all was calm again!

New Year's Day, we went for a walk along the Bude Canal.  Nellie Dean got angry in the car and wanted to go home, so we drove her back to the house. I felt she wanted me to have some time with my husband, but I said she mustn't think we don't want her to come with us. We walked on the moor quickly with the dog instead and when we got back mum asked why she hadn't wanted to come. Crying. "Must be Alzheimer's!" she said, so I returned with her to the moor for another 5 minute walk.

Always ask a person with memory loss for their help instead of telling them what you want them to do!

Nellie Dean says I won't let her go to Surrey. She remembers hearing that there was a care home near my sister, Sal. I said I would investigate for her, but she then denied she has said it at all. For a change I was the one who felt confused!

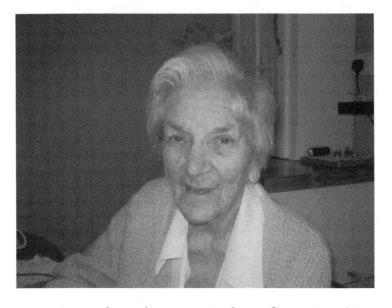

You can see the change in her face in this photo – she looks more tired and is struggling to keep smiling.

Mum was convinced that her tablets were making her ill and, again, appointments at the hospital were a nightmare!

17 times I was asked, one day, why Mum should have tablets at all as she felt so well.

8.30am - just awake – I said she needed to take her "fasting" tablet – She said she would not take it, as her tummy was bad, so she was going to prove a point that it was the tablet causing it. I said - as it was only once a week - therefore it couldn't be the tablet that was the cause - so she took it. It must have been the right answer for once!!

I ran a sink of warm water for her wash and offered help. *"I can manage"* She said. She got dressed without her much loved woolly vest –so I helped her to dress. She said the night tablet had doped her up – not having one again! Couldn't eat dinner.

Said I had *"stitched her up."*

Confusion plays havoc. It is the result of losing connections in the brain and not your loved one trying to be difficult. Heightened confusion could also be due to a Urine Infection.

# Chapter 8

## *TREASURE AND REFLECTIONS*

I was always picking up discarded pennies and Mum wanted so much to find one too! It was treasure! She bent down to pick one up, but she was mortified to realise it was simply a blob of discarded chewing gum. We laughed together and the next time I saw a coin on the ground, I made sure she saw it too. I guided her to it so she could "find" it. Nellie Dean was delighted!

When we were young and on a holiday at the coast, Mum made a game for us kids. On the beach we would all search for cowrie shells. Very difficult to spot! I seemed to be lucky on each of our holidays and spent many wonderful days scouring the sands for them! Her ashes were eventually scattered on our favourite beach in Devon. The first time I re-visited "our" beach after mum passed away, I was just walking with my head down and not particularly looking, and there in front of me was the tiniest of cowrie shells! I have it to this day and it's the best shell I have ever found! I truly believe Mum put it there for me to find and was walking beside me that day.

The day mum passed away a white feather wafted down in front of me. I picked it up as a sign that all was well. Some people say that a white feather is sent by an angel. I like to feel that is true.

We discovered Mum had collected mirrors in the garage of her old house. She was superstitious and could not throw them away even if they were broken!

In the old days, mirrors were very expensive and there is a superstition that you will have 7 years' bad luck if you destroy or break one. They are also said to reflect the soul.

After several years of dementia Nellie Dean decided she hated mirrors and would not use them to comb her hair, or look at herself, which we thought strange, being, at one time, she had collected them. I realised, that when she looked in the mirror – which indeed was on her bathroom wall - she didn't see herself but an old lady staring back at her. She would never look in a mirror again.

She would often say to me that she didn't have a mirror in her bathroom, although there was one there all the time and another hung in her bedroom.

I had no idea that people with dementia perceive themselves young and see their reflection in a mirror as an old person they don't know - even an intruder. We should be careful when placing mirrors.

I watched as Mum became Nellie Dean. She was different to the person I had known all my life. I had to tread carefully if I was to look after this lady I was no longer sure of. I had to learn to care for someone, whose reactions to me I was no longer familiar with, or certain of. Like many other carers, I tried my best. I was learning, but not fast enough.

I took some more courses on communicating, safeguarding and human rights. I was hungry for learning and the internet provided plenty for me to study.

On the internet, I had met many people who were in the same situation as myself and I had read several books about coping with Alzheimer's and related topics. It certainly helped me to understand the reasons behind mum's behaviour.

Through all the repetitiveness; the shadowing and the stubbornness, my life was consumed with doing my best to appease. Trying to find any time for myself and my husband was a problem. I now know that many marriages cannot withstand having an in-law with dementia in their home. I have even heard people say: "It's me or your mum/or dad" to their spouse. It's a hard choice but one that leads to divorce in many cases.

Many times siblings refuse to help or say they can't handle caring and this too will break many families up.

My sister ran a farm shop and her days were spent feeding and tending her animals. My brother was still living in Norway. So, you see, there really was no one else able to look after mum. When mum came to live with us we had no idea what dementia was or how it would change our lives.

Shopping was a nightmare!! Nellie Dean said her shoes were awful and she could not walk in them, but would decline new ones as soon as we entered a shoe shop. I became good at guessing her shoe type and ordered from a catalogue instead. If we were out shopping for clothing I was unable to convince Nellie Dean that she needed new things. Her wardrobe contained 2 dresses, one skirt and a few blouses!

Furniture buying was even more difficult!

It took 3 months to choose the wardrobes Mum liked at a local store. They looked lovely in cream and were an expensive choice, but they were the only ones she wanted. They arrived on Monday and were duly built by my lovely husband. By Thursday morning, the wardrobes appeared white and hurt her eyes. They became a focus for her anger. I was going to paint them blue but decided that would probably upset her too. I was treading on eggshells most of the time!!

Mum would never dream of speaking out, on her own behalf, but Nellie Dean would shout and rant about all sorts of things that displeased her. Not wishing to buy new clothes when needed and visits to the doctor or dentist, were the main cause of consternation to her. I guessed at clothes and bought them for her. I also discovered that the best way to keep appointments at doctor's surgery was to tell her it was an annual check-up the doctor had asked for! Changing into clean clothes was not what Nellie Dean wanted to do! She would often say: *"So long as my body and mind are clean, I don't care what people think!"* I couldn't argue with her but I needed to come to terms with how people saw her and how it reflected on me. I knew dress was not seen as important in dementia care, but I also became cunning. As Nellie Dean got into bed each night, I would quickly throw her clothes out of sight and put new ones out for the morning. By the time morning came Nellie Dean assumed they were her clothes from the day before! I made the mistake of buying her a new pink cardigan from her favourite retailer. I came to realise she hated pink as well as red! She said it was not hers. It had someone else's name on it.

"*Damart*" was the person it belonged to!

I even became a seamstress, altering a charity shop size 22 dress down to a size 10, as it was the same as the one she always loved the best and wore day after day!

I became psychologist, seamstress and detective!

# Chapter 9

## *CUDDLES*

Mum was never a very cuddly person, but Nellie Dean loved a cuddle! I needed the cuddles too!

I recall a long time ago, when I had young children, the chimney on our house caught fire. My father was on the roof spraying water down the chimney, when he called to mum, asking her to go *back inside the house* and listen to see if she could hear the crackling noises stop! My children were sitting on a wall in the back garden cuddling their teddies and other precious toys, watching all this unfold! My daughters have never forgotten the episode which, thankfully, ended well!

Back in Cornwall, mum continued to sketch. I was surrounded by her drawings, mainly of trees and landscapes. How she loved this wonderful world! So I asked if she would like some of them framed. Jo at the pub, who always treated mum as special, gave us a window space for mum's very own solo exhibition. Mum was delighted! Proceeds from any sales at £5 - £10 were donated to a dementia charity.

Too late, I discovered mum thought the proceeds would go to the Children's Trust in Surrey, which was a charity close to her heart. Not wanting to upset her, I explained that the money would go to some very young children who have dementia too.

I discovered the need to become very inventive as a coping mechanism! I didn't always get things right but I was learning to forgive myself.

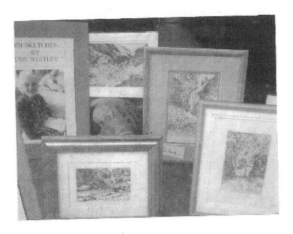
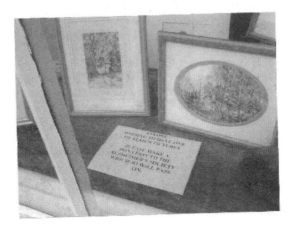

The solo art exhibition

One day we were driving to the hospital in Truro for an appointment and we were hungry. But we also need to stop for a loo break. A red and yellow sign was looming on the horizon, so I called in for a desperate comfort break and – big mistake – I bought 2 plain burgers. Oops! Her face was a picture! She took the top off the bun and peered inside! "Well!" she said and "What is it?" I creased up laughing and she too saw the funny side for she had never seen such a thing in her life before!! It certainly wasn't for eating, however hungry she was!

We might only drive for a few minutes and the familiar: "It's a long way" would ring several times in my ears. I think I counted 14 times on a trip to the hospital one day and 16 times asking why she should take her tablets for cancer as she felt quite well. Incredibly mum was coping with cancer *and* dementia.

I decided, for sanity, to make a game of the repetition and silently counted the times the words were repeated, or I would have aborted the appointment!

So on the next trip to the hospital, we sang all the way instead and avoided the burger bar!

I also discovered that if I said "It's a long way" first, for some reason, it stopped My Nellie Dean from repeating the words again.

Repetition is a common symptom and you need to find ways of coping!

# Chapter 10

## *OUR NEW FRIENDS*

"SPOOKY"

A stray cat chose us! Spooky by name and spooked by nature! The cat took around 6 months to sum up the courage to come in the house!

Nellie Dean did battle with the cat, however! Spooky was not used to being stroked and would lash out. They were a good match for each other, as it gave the danger mum craved and she admired the little cat's independence. It frightened me to death and I kept the medical cabinet close by!!! Spooky made us her forever home, where she was allowed to be as wild as she liked!

Nellie Dean decided her bedroom window would stay open all night so Spooky could get in during the winter months. A huge row ensued, with Nellie Dean refusing to close her window. Later that week I called for help from a social care visitor who talked to mum and came to an agreement with her, that her window should be locked, as the snow was getting in the room. However, mum didn't remember the conversation or talking about the cat getting in the window.

So Spooky became a bedfellow when Nellie Dean went to sleep!

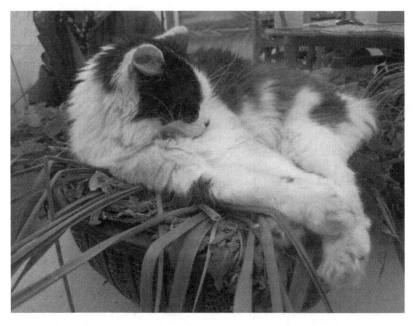

Spooky liked to help with the hanging baskets!

"HOLLY"

We were given a small Jack Russell dog, to comfort mum, by a neighbour who could no longer keep a dog.  Holly proved to be more of a comfort than I could ever be. Holly would not answer back and expected nothing more than cuddles and biscuits. She would sit on Nellie Dean's lap in the car and there was no better prescription. Holly was born to make people laugh! On the day we picked her up she jumped over the backseat and was then unable to jump back again, due to the incline of the rear seat! I looked in my mirror to see a bouncing up and down Holly – just like the dog in the John Smith's advert!! From that first day, Holly had made us laugh. She had to come everywhere with us including to memory café, where she proved to be an excellent "Pets As Therapy" dog and was more than welcome.

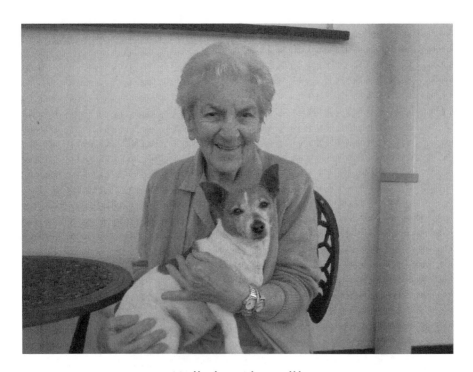

Holly loved us all!

Animals have a very special bond with people who have dementia.

# Chapter 11

## *SINGING IN THE RAIN*

We would sing!

If it was a bright day, the choice was "Sunny Skies are Here Again" or "You are my Sunshine"

Rainy weather brought on "Somewhere over the Rainbow" and "I'm singing in the Rain". If we were stuck behind a van, it was: "My old Man Said Follow the Van" or even "Postman Pat". If we passed a church we would sing "The Bells Are Ringing for Me and My Gal", and so on. I felt quite proud of myself having learnt all the words to songs that were before my time. I don't think mum would have appreciated "Yellow Submarine" somehow!!!

Then, of course, we would always sing "There's an old mill by the Stream" - whatever the weather!

Our heaven was driving around the lanes. The place she felt safe. Her "Home" not *at* home, wherever that was to her now – but just OUT, going places. No pressure. The fun of singing songs and the uplift of being able to remember the words when I forgot them. A familiar place - "our place". A favourite phrase was "I've seen that tree before!" It comforted her to imagine she still knew her way around but, oh boy! There were a lot of trees she had seen before!! We spent many days out and about.

Sometimes when out, I was a little worried if Nellie Dean got out of the car in the car park. She could not remember which car was mine and no longer had any road sense. She repeatedly confirmed to me that the green one was my car but - ! - There were many green cars!

Driving along there were always snacks! Chocolate; fish and chips or fruit and always the cardboard pot of fresh orange. Most of

Nellie Dean's drinks were then taken in the car on our trips out. She loved hot tea but, at the care home, it was never provided hot enough for her otherwise she might have burnt her mouth. Health and Safety, you see. Well, she didn't burn her mouth! She never drank more than a sip from each cup because it was not hot! A sweet taste pervaded her mouth every time she tried to drink and she convinced herself that the carers were forgetting she didn't take sugar. No-one ever asked her why she was not drinking. It was simply assumed that she had forgotten to drink it. In her room there was always fresh orange, water and other cold drinks, but that delicious cuppa eluded her.

I think it strange that no-one thinks to ask a person with dementia why they do something – after all it is simple to ask!

## WHERE IS HOME?

After living with my husband and me for a few years Mum said:

*"I am just having a 2 week holiday here."*

I replied that all her things were here and we go to art class and garden club.

Nellie Dean could not explain where Home" was to me. When I asked her if it was Surrey or London she simply said "no". She was certainly feeling lost inside all the time.

I learnt that "Home" for Nellie Dean was not a physical place but a feeling of safety and familiarity which was difficult to find in her world of dementia.

We carried on visiting memory cafes during this time. I kept a copy of a poem written at the Memory Cafe by Nellie Dean: "*Water:*

*Water, water, rushing down, from the sky so very high. It's making puddles on the ground. Little children splashing around. How they love a rainy day so they can go paddling on the plane. The ground's so wet, it's such a treat (and so she gets all wet)*"

Mum had always loved children and particularly babies. They were all precious to her, having lost her first born. All babies were special but, at the grand age of 92, she had not held a baby for many years.

The Memory Café in Launceston provided the joy and a friend who was grandma to twins.

She had no qualms about letting mum hold her babies and even give them their bottle feed. So special!

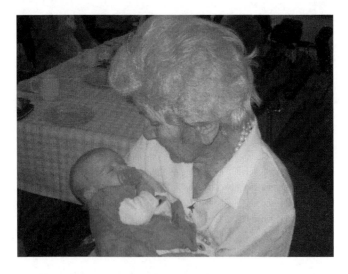

Ever since my father passed away my mother had hoped for a partner to waltz again with her. Many times, at the Memory Cafes, opportunities presented themselves and yes – she could still waltz – even teaching a line dancer to waltz in the middle of her routine!!

There was never anyone but my father for mum! No man could ever waltz as well as he did!

For years I had watched them waltzing together – sweeping across the dance floor as though they were the only couple in the whole world! Unbeknown to them, I was sitting on the side-line with tears running down my face! I was so proud that they were *my* mum and dad! When the time arrived that Nellie Dean could no longer walk very well at all, I would hum the tune to the Blue Danube and like magic she could dance. "One, two, three, one, two three", she would repeat to me as we danced along.

For months she was steadier on her feet if she was dancing, rather than walking. We took part in a short Memory Walk and three quarters of the way round mum could not move another step. I could not carry her, so I decided to hum The Blue Danube and we both danced to the finishing line together!

Memory cafes were a lifeline to Nellie Dean and to me! The cafés gave stability in a topsy-turvy world for us both.

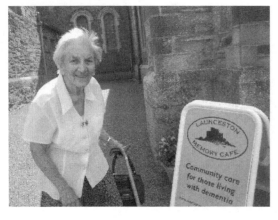

We had arrived at the café one week, as usual, and needed to visit the ladies room first. I had assisted Nellie Dean with her underwear and, while she washed her hands, I heard her ask: "Would you like me to help you now?" "I am managing just fine!!" I replied, trying very hard not to laugh out loud. She was always so very thoughtful of others! Or, perhaps, it was her way to tell me that it is difficult to allow another person to assist with personal care?

Try not to do too much for the person with memory loss. It is a natural reaction when caring but better if the person achieves themselves.

## PASTRY

I have many special memories such as the many times we made pastry together. Mum would mix and I would make. Each time she would tell me only to use my fingertips and very cold water. Mum always had cold hands, (warm heart!) but she always had to run cold water over her fingers just to make sure they were as cold as possible. She always made the best pastry!

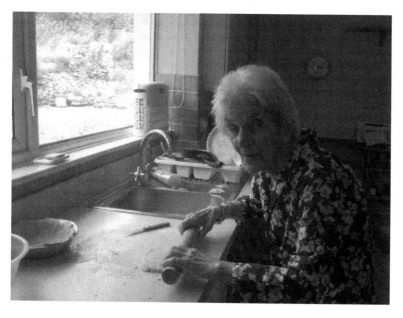

Mum picked up the rolling pin and rolled out the pastry.

The pie was made and I put a wash cloth for her to clean the worktop. However, when I turned around My Nellie Dean was happily ensconced, rolling out the dishcloth to perfection! When it was perfect and, without further ado, I placed it carefully on a baking tray and into the oven to cook.

I felt sad that yet another skill was being lost.

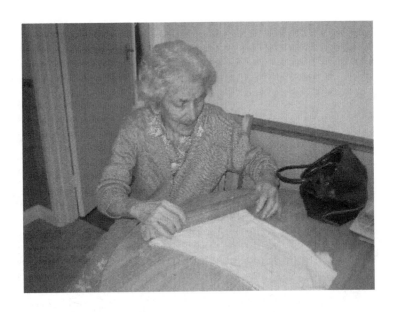

Nellie Dean could still see perfectly without glasses but to her it simply looked like pastry! She was stuck in the joy of the rolling movement, and of being useful. There were always bits of pastry over and these were the "waste not want not" bits. They were carefully made into jam tarts with home-made blackberry jelly. Making dog biscuits became easier to cope with when unidentified objects began to appear in the pastry!

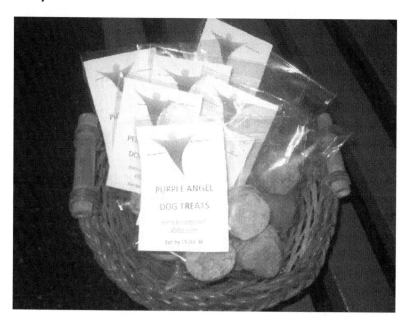

Once there were 5 jam tarts on a plate and for each one I was asked "Oh Jam tarts, my favourite! Could I have one?"

I don't suppose it hurt to eat them all!

"The Queen of Hearts, she ate some tarts"!

This is typical of dementia where the person cannot remember recent events even for a few minutes and the brain can also compensate with actions that appear to us to be strange but not to them.

All care was gone and Nellie Dean danced in the centre of Launceston town with Norrms. The band were playing and the day was jolly!

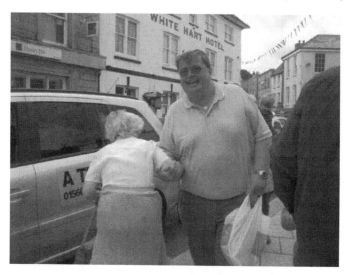

I could not help with the waltzing! My father always said I had two left feet and he was right! Eventually Nellie Dean lost her balance, forgot the steps, and would never dance again. We continued to walk together for quite a while even with a wheelchair at times.

Balance and gait are affected with dementia. Emotional responses seem to remain long after events which explains why people never forget the way you make them feel.

Gardening kept us busy much of the time.

We planted seedlings and watched them grow. Potting on was dodgy, as Nellie Dean was never sure if the green bit went in the pot first, and I would effect a rescue when she wasn't looking!

Her favourite job was to sweep the poly-tunnel and she repeatedly told me that the best gardeners kept a clean ship!

Weeding, she said, was a waste of time!

Life was far too precious for that!

I still weed the garden today but her words ring in my mind and I agree it *is* a waste of time as they always grow back again!!

Picking fruit together was another job to be done which mum enjoyed. She never seemed to notice the scratches from the gooseberry bushes and was determined not to leave a berry on the bush!

We would drive miles looking for blackberries. Mum had been very fond of making blackberry jelly each year with the harvest. She would to pick the berries with the aid of her trusty walking stick to hook down the briars. She was still able to wash the jars but, of course, I had to pour the hot jelly for her.

I am left with fond memories each year when I keep up the family tradition. We also made cakes and potted up a few small jars for sale at the memory café.

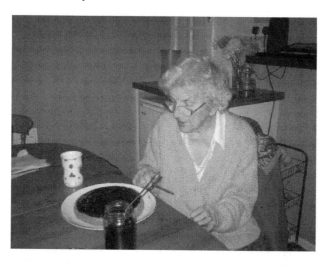

Decorating cakes with blackberry jelly

# Chapter 12

## *BEHIND CLOSED DOORS*

2nd January: "I've had a heart attack in the night" 8.30am – "Do you know I've had a near death experience?" Me: "Yes. This tablet will make you feel better soon". To this day I don't know what happened to her that night, but five minutes later she was back to her busy self again.

Next day 6am: Wandering up and down the hallway. Woke me up. I called out "I'm still here" and she went back to bed. 6.30 Nellie Dean shouted *"Are you in?"* Just wanted a cuppa so I got up and made the tea. 7am I sat with her with tea then she said she was going back to bed. It seemed as though I was not allowed to have a lay in! Went to mum. Gone to bed. Tea half drunk. She then got up again and I asked if she would like help with a nice shower. "I'm not dirty" she said.

I told her I never said she was! She started to wash and dress. It soon became clear she mistakenly thought we were going out and I was waiting for her. I showered me. I asked her to sit with her feet up for a while, as they were swollen and hurting, and I would bring breakfast to her. One minute later she got up to get her bag. Hrmph! I told her to sit down again.  5 mins later she was in the kitchen to help me? I said I was getting breakfast as fast as I could and asked if she would go and sit down again. 8.30 I took breakfast in to her. Days of wandering – in and out, early in the morning, then going to her bed saying she is *"dying", "legs hurt/breathing so bad"*. Said she didn't want to go to sleep as she may not wake up again. She has a bell to ring for me, but can't remember to ring it. Said she won't have a Zimmer frame as there is nothing wrong with her. I purchased a circulation booster, but won't try it. Later, I did manage to get her to try it out and it at least worked well to keep her sitting down!  I was very worried all the time for her swollen legs, as she would not sit for any length of time at all with them up.  She kept on walking, even though she accepted my help to go back to her chair, then 5 minutes later she was up again. Breathing shallow, face a good colour. Went to the toilet on her own. I offered help to wash – No. "I'm OK". Cold in the night (will not have heating on and wants window open again – and it is snowing!) On the toilet, I took her a gown. "I bet I'm constipated now" "OK – we'll have some prunes". I asked if she felt better – "Oh yes, I'm fine". Because she knew she had Alzheimer's and, from time to time, she was very distressed – she cried often.  I tried to help her, but it made it worse.  I told her everything was OK and she said I don't know what it's like.  I tried to get her to rest, but won't sit for even 2 minutes – she truly believed she sits all day. She wanted to know how this all ends – I couldn't speak. (I must say next time: "everyone is different"). Mum has many temper outburst she doesn't recall. Blank hours/days. Follows me and wants to know where I am all day – though I am here. Very jealous of my friends – the one or two I have left now. Mum loved to wash up and do the ironing but Nellie Dean said *SHE* was *MY* slave! Then she was leaving again to work in a home in Surrey. A 10 minute memory for things said or done. No concept of day or time. Compulsively going through pictures and papers, trying to remember – bagging up paperwork and empty crisp packets and used envelopes during the night. Accusing me of taking/moving things. Can't follow a television program, read a book or sketch anymore. Very tired all day.  I too am becoming exhausted and I am lost.

One Wednesday night I started thinking and could not sleep.

Shadowing, repetition, constant attention, no time for me. I can't go out anywhere on my own. She is fussing, crying all the time, depressed and needs nursing care for her now swollen legs. Constantly wanting to know where I am and what I am doing. I feel emotionally harassed. Being followed all day. No time with my husband. My friends are no good and Nellie Dean doesn't want to live with me. I must not believe what Alzheimer's is saying. She walks from 8am till 10.30pm. She won't rest her legs or go to bed until I say I am going to tuck down. I worry about her. I know dad has been calling her to him, but somehow she must suffer longer still. She knows we have been out together but can't remember what we did. Such precious memories to her and they do not stay with her, for even one day. I tell her she has plenty of old memories to cherish but she's distressed realising again (for the first time) that her memory is going. I forgot to cuddle her tonight but still pray that God will take her.  Will she eventually be alone when he does? Will it be at night with no-one by her side? How unfair this disease is.

Alzheimer's makes her think she's able to do anything and everything, especially the things I do. She is living her life through me. I feel like a surrogate brain. She is on her feet all day but has no idea she is doing that. Only sits for meals. Backwards and forwards "Where's Jane?" Many times over. If I dare to go out for an hour on my own, my husband gets the 3rd degree, and she doesn't believe him when he tells her where I am. She then goes to a neighbour to confirm that she is not supposed to be with me. Whatever I do, she wants to do too. It's wearing herself out and me too.  Doesn't remember what she just did so thinks she hasn't done anything. I take her for a walk and she immediately goes for another walk because she doesn't remember she has been. Says she knits/draws but doesn't. Doesn't accept she is 89 and just like others of that age and will not visit the age concern coffee morning as "they are all old".

I can't even have a bath to relax, or go to the toilet, without she wants to join me. No relaxation at all as she is in and out, but won't sit with us. (Nellie Dean would decline joining my husband and me to sit and watch TV in the evenings. I didn't realise at the time that she could no longer follow a story and therefore, to her, we were absorbed by something we were looking at that she could no longer understand). She excused herself, saying she wanted us to have some time on our own, but the truth was she was unable to admit that she could no longer follow a story on TV or read a book. Nellie Dean was in denial throughout the whole of her illness. Nellie Dean was never cold and always professed she didn't need a coat or jacket.

Nellie Dean had frequent nosebleeds and one that I remember well lasted several hours in the middle of the night. She called me to help and could not understand what was happening to her. Was it cancer? A tumour? Where was all the blood coming from? She was frightened and wanted to know. Her carpet and bed were covered in blood and after a couple of hours the nose bleed subsided and I cleared the room up.

Thankfully, dementia kicked in and on this occasion was welcome visitor as she forgot all about the episode and went back to sleep – the whole episode completely and thankfully erased. I, of course, was by then wide awake!

The cooker had been disconnected long ago due to Nellie Dean nearly setting our house on fire. Then the microwave had to go too when she cooked a cup of coffee for 3 hours instead of 3 minutes. The door of the refrigerator was often left ajar and water seeped on to the kitchen floor when it defrosted.

We were frightened Nellie Dean would slip, so that went from her kitchen too.

One of the worst trials of dementia must surely be the loss of life skills and needing full time care.

Early evening I needed to pick something up from the local shop. I was gone 10 minutes and came back to find Nellie Dean wandering in the dark and frosty garden outside the house, dressed only in her nightie. Another evening I am trying to keep some form of normality by going to a garden club meeting. Nellie Dean wants to know where I am and won't believe what my husband tells her, so she goes to ask a neighbour. Because Nellie Dean doesn't remember for more than a few minutes, I can no longer leave her. She is becoming disorientated if I go out at all. Repetitive – where am I –facts all wrong and thinks she should go with me. Constantly edgy and worrying. Very sad and lonely. Won't do what I ask her and doesn't rest day or night. I am running short of ideas to keep the peace.

Fri night: not much sleep for either of us and Nellie Dean is tired in the day. Suggested herbal tablets might help her sleep.

Saturday night: with mum at midnight spitting into sink but I cannot discover why. Perhaps she was feeling sick. Bad day Sunday. Sunday night no sleep, nose bleed, back to bed at 7.30am. Up again 5 minutes later. Offered to help her wash, back to bed and then up again. No wonder she is tired and I am absolutely worn to a frazzle. Perhaps she has a urine infection which can make a person even more confused and agitated?

Monday: 7.30am Nellie Dean said she had not slept. She went back to bed, saying she is dying.  Helped her into bed – leg hurt. 7.35am, got up again. She won't try taking some herbs to help her sleep (i.e. a light sleep aid). Won't put legs up but they hurt. She certainly won't have a sleeping tablet either. I can't do any more for her. She refuses to go to a care home for me to get a break.

Then the Hairdresser arrived and she was fine. Afterwards, she became angry again for no reason I can imagine – said she would go to Surrey to a home. Nellie Dean was very hateful to me and my patience was at an end. I rang Sal to find out what it was like at the home near her, but it didn't sound good. Nellie Dean told Sal she was going to live with a neighbour in Surrey. Crying.

She said the care home I took her to for some respite was a lovely place. She had no idea how abusive she had been when we drove to the home. I tried to take her again the following week, but by the time I had driven her there, I was more stressed trying to get some respite than not! Wednesday: Up and awake so I took tea in and 10mins later Nellie Dean was back to sleep. Later we went for a ride out in the car and walk.

Lunchtime she went to bed to sleep, so tired, had 5 mins and up again. Legs swollen. No feet up and so it went on.

5th Dec 2009: A drive in the car to my sister's house for the 40th art group party. The art group had been her whole life and she was an honorary member. Mum said she wanted to go so I had made arrangements. Then: *"Don't want to go. Want to die. Don't want tablets"*. I was in need of respite but nevertheless, worried whether Mum would be happy at my Sister's for a few days.

The day before the party – Mum said she was dying – called me *"wicked"*. I gently drove her to my sister's house in Surrey, whereupon she said she was looking forward to seeing her other daughter. Later she said she didn't want to leave her cat or go to any party as her bottom teeth were loose. In the morning, my sister woke her to go to market and same again – said she was ill. When my sister had gone to market, leaving mum behind with a nephew to look after her, Nellie Dean then phoned to ask where everyone had gone – why was she left on her own?

When mum was back home with me, my sister phoned: She said Mum was not happy living with me. She doesn't like the atmosphere and doesn't like Cornwall. She wants to buy a house in Surrey or have a caravan and live with my sister.

I was told a different story: Mum said she was alone for hours at my sister's house and felt useless with nothing to do. Said it was nice to be home with me. Said she had made scotch eggs and been out delivering farm produce with my sister. The following day Mum said she didn't want to live with my sister. She was bored sitting alone sketching in the garden. Felt redundant, as she couldn't help on the farm with anything, so just talked to the customers in the farm shop but felt she was being a nuisance.

If Nellie Dean was confused then so was I! Despite all this I still felt that mum was so brave. It must be so very hard to be losing not just all her memories but everything she had ever known.

Nellie Dean cannot understand she is 89 or that she is ill. A friend offered to be with mum for a day or an evening to give me a break, but I can't ask as she was hurtful once before and I can't put this on to friends. I felt a failure. Everything I did mum had to do too. When I was given a small gardening job across the road, I tried to explain that I get paid for the gardening and because of her infirmity, she cannot come to work with me.

The shadowing seemed to me like a fear of missing out on something and insecurity. I tried to understand. Nellie Dean wanted to come to social meetings in the evenings and go everywhere I went. Pub nights out, friends for coffee and shopping were all out of the question for me now. She could not understand that it was too much for her. One evening she thought my husband and I had gone out and left her but were only sitting in the lounge.

As Nellie Dean reached further into her world of dementia I found we had to adapt. A trip to the seaside presented its own problems as Nellie Dean began to strip off. Everything! How could I even begin to explain to her that revealing all Mother Nature gives you is wrong?!

Well, for once, I was confounded! I began to dress her, much to her annoyance, and decided to avoid the beach in future!

Typical day: Up 9am breakfast. To Widemouth Bay - trip out till 12. Then Ironing, Singing at the local care home, out in the garden, dinner, walking around.

Sat down for just 5 minutes. It was 10pm. Nellie Dean was not tired.

Sunday: 9am had breakfast, walked at a local beauty spot. 11.30 had lunch, 12 went to a car boot sale with me and stood till dinner time at 6pm. On her feet all day till 10.45 only going to bed when I did. Constant walking and threats to me: I'm too clean; my friends are no good for me; don't like Cornwall and how great my brother and sister are. Following me – *"Where's Jane?* She doesn't accept she has Alzheimer's and blames me although she will use "I have dementia" when she feels like it! Bothering neighbours and going off walking up the road so I follow at a distance to keep eye on her. Seems to be looking for psychological help with her dementia but there is none available. My friends are no good and I am *"just like Dad - pig headed!"*

Nellie Dean will not have clean clothes or her pills for her heart. Will not recognise she came to live with me because she needed help and says she came as *I was not happy*(!) Says I have made her lazy but still can't manage to do anything for herself. Says she can live on her own but cannot sort out an appointment or make a cup of tea. I can't do anything right.

Wednesday: Take her home from art – too ill to go out to a special dinner. There followed 2 weeks of hell, dying, heart attacks and sore gums. The doctor said she was as fit as a fiddle and gave sleeping tablets for me to use as required. Dentist said nothing wrong with gums although teeth are a problem so need new ones. (That would have been a whole new ball-game!) Problem: won't stop putting teeth in and then thinks she has mouth cancer because her gums hurt, so I took her teeth away. She was angry with me all week, although not over the teeth, and I lost my composure! Sad to say, I told her she was being a c-o-w to me. I told her I was doing my best. Things were better for next 2 days till Thurs. Woke with tea at 8.15am – straight away said she had a bad night, fast heartbeat and sore throat. Said her tummy felt funny too. I put Holly our dog on the bed with her in the hope she would stay in bed and said I thought she could have a cold.

Thus our days went by in a muddle of confused emotions.

January 2010: Nellie Dean puts her coat on, as I go out each time, and wants a walk herself even though her legs will not carry her. Doesn't understand where I/we have gone even for 15 mins and gets confused.

Sadly she is no longer able to keep herself occupied. She truly believes she still knits, paints and does gardening but doesn't do these things any longer and can't settle unless I give her a task. Life is sad for her and for me. I feel her life is no longer her own but belongs to this demon of a disease.

One day we walked with the help of her wheelchair but she wanted to sleep. She was tired and breathless – unable to walk many steps. We had coffee in Bude and I pushed the wheelchair back to the car. Still breathless and tired. At home, we ate lunch then Mum wanted to sleep. 1pm went to go for a sleep – No!  1.30pm: said again going to sleep – No! 1.36pm going for a rest but went out in the garden. 2pm going for rest. 2.15pm came out into the garden. I took her back indoors for a sleep as she was tearful and confused. I was becoming stressed. "Burnout" was looming.

On the Monday we went to her Cognitive Stimulation Class - something she loved to do despite not being able to understand any of the quizzes and puzzles; Tuesday she was tired after having an ECG. That afternoon she was unwell, depressed and tearful. Tablets for her heart are still a problem and often they are refused.

The repetitive behaviour, the shadowing. Following me from morning till evening, sometimes seeking me out at night time too, was beginning to take its toll on my health. There was an occasion I slipped away for a bath and Nellie Dean asked my husband where I had gone. She said she could get in the bath with me! Late nights, dealing with nosebleeds and incessant paper collecting during the dark hours, were having a big effect.

We visited the dentist several times with the aim of getting loose teeth pulled out. Nellie Dean was not eating very well and often saying how her mouth hurt. Each time we arrived at the dentist she denied having a problem and wouldn't let the dentist do what was needed. Eventually, after wasted appointments the matter was taken up at a best interest meeting and it was decided nothing should be done.

Her false teeth often went missing and she would tell me she had thrown them away by mistake. I spent hours looking through the bins and even down the toilet for them!

Dealing with bills, medication, hospital visits, cancelling repeat charity donations on her bank statements, dentist, chiropodist and hairdressers. Then there was my life – I was unable to have a job or contribute to our family life. I missed visits to my children, who lived far away, and having less time for my husband made me feel sad.

I couldn't sleep well. I woke several times a night. Thoughts of her getting worse and not knowing me anymore. My own health is beginning to fail with episodes of anxiety and stress. I became ill and reached what the professionals call "burn out".

I was asked to sign paperwork stating that I would no longer care for my mother. That hurt me deeply.

There was no support to keep mum by my side nor any chance of respite.

The care home assessor said she saw through Nellie Dean's protective layer "She's very good at covering it up" she said to me. But Nellie Dean wasn't being deceitful (God forbid! She had taught me not to tell lies all my childhood!) She was merely putting on a brave face and hiding her problems, knowing full well that she had dementia and using her only defence to keep it from the professionals and from me too. .

Imaginative – Yes! Stubborn – Yes! But, despite all, still so very loved for how she lived and loved us all! Dementia could not win.

People with dementia are good at compensating for their memory loss.

I was being threatened with going to Sally or a *"bloody"* care home.

Nellie Dean sure likes *clearing the air* with a row.

She said Spooky, the cat, is her only friend in Cornwall and persistently asks my husband to move a sofa to another room for her. (He moved it twice already!)

She cannot accept the doctor in Cornwall — she doesn't know him.

Says she will go and live with a neighbour in Surrey or get a job at a care home and stay there.

Note from mum which she tore up:

*"Thanks a Bunch" "Once again I have fallen for it. I'd no idea she was getting rid of me again in the Old Folks Home! I can stay in my own garden - I really*

*need to get back to Surrey. How I wish I'd talk to Sally about going back. I must go to the doctor and get a bill of health! I can't imagine why I am so gullible!! That's the worst of being so trusting."*

Exhausting activity – never on my own and I seem to be getting mentally abused by mum. Almost as though she thinks it is my fault that she is ill.

Sometimes dementia will give a person a different view of "socially acceptable behaviour" and unexpected emotions are common. Frontotemporal dementia, in particular, can exhibit a change in socially inappropriate behaviour, lack of inhibition, concentration and speech difficulties and abrupt mood changes

Chapter 13

## *THE CARE HOME*

The sad day came when I had to admit that if I wanted to continue to look after Nellie Dean, then the only way would be to place her in care so I could get some rest and recovery myself.

A friend had warned me that when she was a carer she became so stressed that one day she simply walked out of the door, with no coat on, and ended up on a park bench. She said I should not leave it too late to place mum in care or get some help. I took head of her words.

Nellie Dean chose her care home from several we had visited together holding singalongs. It was not the home I would have chosen for her but I needed to listen. It was homely, she said.

To my sister she wrote: *"I am going into a nursing home. I think it is Wednesday - not sure. It is 6 o'clock this morning and I am wide awake. Cat's still asleep but has been up for her breakfast. Jane has arranged a visit to a local home for Alzheimer's patients - whosoever they are.... Now it's my turn. I will let you know how I get on. Mum."*

On top of everything, the social care assessor decided I had defrauded the Government by taking out an investment, which meant the council could only use the interest and not the capital. Seriously? I had no idea how those things worked.

Shortly after being placed into a care home Mum became ill with shingles and had a painful rash. She was in a great deal of pain and I felt that it was all my fault. Mum could not remember why she was bedridden – thinking she had suffered a heart attack or fall - so I wrote a note and pinned it to her bedside cabinet saying: "You have shingles and will be well again soon"

A request from Mum for a hot water bottle for comfort was denied as Health and Safety rules did not permit the use of them. Even a microwave bottle was not acceptable. That was tough and my heart sank. I left a note saying *"Remember this! I love you xxx from Jane"* (Later mum changed the note to read from Elsie to Jane.)

Thus we began to write notes to each other.

In the care home mum would constantly write notes. She would practice her own signature, poems she cherished, days of the week and so on. She was trying to hold on but knew her memory was failing. Despite her outward denial, she knew deep down that she really did have Alzheimer's.

We went through the usual: "What's your name" which I was expecting but it was still a tough thing to hear. From that day on I would greet her with: "Hi mum! It's your daughter Jane!" I was not prepared to let her forget me again.

Some days she would become angry at the slightest thing I said and I realised if I was to keep my mother, and her love for me, I would need to accept whatever she said without question. I was told I should "jump into mum's world" but I had to completely re-learn my world. I had to change my responses and even forget some of the things she taught me - such as always telling the truth. I was prepared when Nellie Dean forgot my name but I was not prepared when she said "I could kill you". I shouted in disbelief: "Don't you ever say that again" and immediately regretted letting dementia win. I must have evoked emotions, as it never did happened again.

As a new mother myself, my mother would teach me how to bring up children. One should not say "Because I said so" when a child asks a question. So I tried to explain when Nellie Dean asked me questions. How many times I wanted to say: "because I said so" when she asked me why she should do something she didn't want to do!!!

Asking me if my father was ill or dead, I replied truthfully and just the once, that he was gone and I still missed him dearly. A few months later Nellie Dean told me my father was gone. It had taken a long time for her to process the information and she never mentioned him again.

A cry for comfort needs to be addressed. Just a listening ear or an understanding look can mean so much. Never argue or confront!

Mum had collected all the classics and many books on art. She had a huge library and so I was sad when the day came that she no longer showed any interest. For the same reasons we had to stop looking at family photos. They no longer meant anything to her and, reminding her of her sisters and so on, just made her stressed. It was another reason why music became so important to her. There was no pressure.

She loved to wear her pearl necklaces but one day they became too difficult to undo and she ripped them off. Pearls flew everywhere and she decided she no longer liked to wear any jewellery at all.

At the care home I was asked by other residents' families what to do when visiting. They did not know how to converse or act. After visiting mum every other day of the week for a couple of years, I had found some answers and wrote the following:

# TIPS FOR YOUR VISIT TO A LOVED ONE

Although memories may fade, feelings remain, as does spiritual awareness. Visits can stimulate warm feelings and social interaction can uplift and remain with the person long after your visit.

When you arrive at the care home you may be feeling anxious, guilty or sad - It's completely normal to have these feelings. When you go to visit your loved one it's going to be a little different. He or she won't have been with you all day, and you're no longer his or her 24- hour caregiver. ARRIVE WITH A SMILE – people with dementia tune in to how you are feeling. Wear bright clothes and be positive and encouraging.

Know what time of day is the best time to visit.
As you know from caring for your loved at home, there are certain times of day that he or she is more anxious, upset, and confused.
People with dementia can become more confused later in the day. Your visit can help them to overcome this "sun-downing", as it is called, by keeping their minds active, relaxed and happy.
Most people are tired by late afternoon and the best time

to visit is at least a couple of hours before sun-downing usually arrives.

MAKE SURE THE LIGHT IS NOT BEHIND YOU – People with dementia can have problems seeing you if the light is blaring out behind you and extremes of dark and light can confuse. Eyesight generally becomes more narrowed as we age but is a particular problem for people with dementia who can suffer tunnel vision and it is better if the light is on *your* face so they can see you clearly. If you can, minimise background noise.

FACE THE PERSON and don't shout! USE GENTLE TOUCH BUT BE AWARE THAT SOME MAY NOT LIKE THIS METHOD SO BE CAREFUL HOW YOU USE CONTACT.

MAKE EYE CONTACT AND SPEAK SLOWLY AND CLEARLY. INTRODUCE YOURSELF EACH TIME YOU VISIT. USE SHORT SENTENCES.

WAIT FOR AN ANSWER – PEOPLE WITH DEMENTIA NEED MORE TIME TO PROCESS WORDS. KEEP QUESTIONS SIMPLE AND DON'T ASK IF THE PERSON "REMEMBERS" – It just upsets when a person can't but knows he/she should remember.

TAKE A MAGAZINE, SOME BOOKS OR PHOTOGRAPHS WITH YOU – maybe an item or two to discuss. Singing a favourite song together is invaluable. Share simple jokes together or tell stories. In earlier stages, socialise by visiting a memory café regularly or joining a Cognitive Stimulation class, visiting shops or walking out to keep active and engaged. For later stages, give a soft toy and take some flowers or herbs such as Rosemary or Lavender with you to smell and touch. A fiddle blanket or a doll may be well received too. Favourite songs and music remain with the person till the end of time.

When it is time to leave your loved one, don't mention you are "going home". You will need to think of another thing you have to be doing such as needing to pick up some shopping and let them know you will be back soon. This is a difficult moment for both the visitor and the person who may often ask to "go home". Many residents will not understand they no longer live with a spouse, let alone that they now live in care. You need to foster an understanding of the new world they live in now. Their "home" is often not a physical environment rather a plea for the life they knew before dementia. If you are confronted by a statement you know is not true – just go with the flow as logic is often disrupted with dementia and it is far better to simply agree or say "Tell me about it". Respond to the emotion behind the words.

You may be feeling upset yourself as you leave having seen your loved one deteriorating a little more each time but be assured your visits provide ongoing support and comfort – The details of your visit may be forgotten but the feelings you leave behind will remain.

©Jane Moore    www.purpleangel-global.com

## THE GUILT MONSTER

Yes, here it was. That guilt monster that we all have inside us. I knew there was nothing else to do, but still the monster called on me, time and time again.

## I AM NOT THERE FOR HER

Guilty. While mum's in the care-home I am cooking and thinking that she should be here with me to eat and I feel anxious that she is not getting the food she is used to. I told my guilt demon that, by choice, mum only ate fruit in her own home so would not miss my cooking. Saw Mum cry on Thursday – felt anxious that I am not there to cuddle her – worried for her future, and mine, as she deteriorated. Anxious as to how it would all end and when. Under pressure and told by the care home not to see Mum so often as I looked tired, made me feel sad. I worried over finances both with Social services and my own family.

SURPRISE!

I hid things….. Kit Kats; chocolate; crisps. Comfort stuff!  Just think how you feel when you discover a bar of chocolate in your cupboard put there a month ago and forgot about! Naughty but nice! These things I orchestrated and hid in various places around her room!

We were home every other day and I had the energy to continue. We made pastry again, sang and danced. We moved since mum was living with us so she didn't feel upset or that our house was "her home". We went to several memory cafes and had fun dancing and socialising.  We sang in the car all the time. Each time we returned to the care home mum said: *"Is this where I live?"* It broke my heart every time I left her.

On my own I continually saw her peeling potatoes, gardening and picking fruits with me on a nice sunny day. I was in bed and thinking of my mum in hers at the care home. I felt guilty and weak. Finances were still a worry at home. I tried to think cosy thoughts and tried to relax, but sound sleep eluded me.

On days we were together, I awoke to a first thought: "See Mum today". I discovered that although my life had become a little easier, Nellie Dean's had not. I could not forgive myself.

I arose and walked out into the garden having very lonely, sad thoughts of mum. How I missed her and felt lost without her by my side. I cooked chicken soup for my friend and felt I should be doing this for mum. Her favourite meal. Despite doing my best for her, guilty thoughts pervaded my life and I worried what she was really feeling. I promised myself that there was much I could still do. I would forever be her main carer until the end and I carried on taking her to places, washing her hair and cooking for her. I would buy boxes of tissues, biscuits, yoghurts, comfortable pads, favourite soap and so on. I would take her macaroni cheese and her favourite vegetable stew.

We were together as much as possible, which I know was what she wanted.

Nellie Dean had accumulated so many things. Paintings, in particular, there must have been 50 or more; books – I could not count them all. These were the things most dear to her and we managed to fill her room with memories. A painting she had done of her mother hung opposite her bed. One day she was wandering around looking for her mother. She said she had seen her and asked me where she had gone. I put my hand on mum's heart and said "She is right here with us" and then I pointed to her painting and said how beautiful my grandma was. It seemed to do the trick and she smiled.

Paperwork was everywhere again. It was like a "porridge pot" and carrier bags just seemed to appear filled with sketches, poems, stories, redundant crisp packets and junk mail.

As fast as I cleared it and threw the sticky chocolate papers, so her handbag became full again!

Her handbag went everywhere with her along with a bag of paperwork and panic ensued if either were lost! The carers were always hunting for her bag, her teeth and glasses – sometimes even discovering other people's glasses and belongings in the porridge pot! No-one really appreciates how hard those carers work!

Most care establishments ask that you keep the décor simple but memories must never be discarded lightly. Nellie Dean's comfort was the cherished items that she collected.

# Chapter 14

## *LETTERS*

One morning mum copied out a well-known poem. She wrote:

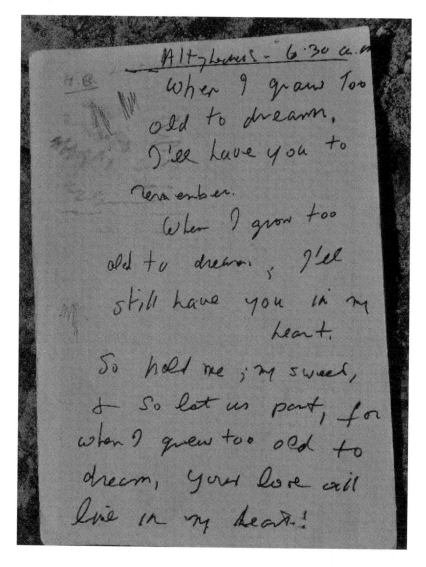

I later found a picture of the heath where my mother and father used to walk together.

On it mum had added the words

*"Please meet there as we used to do"*

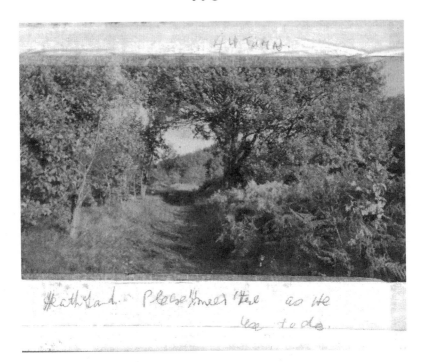

My father, Eddie had always given her 12 pink carnations on their anniversary, since those that she had carried in her wedding bouquet.

After he died I continued to send them on his behalf. She loved the flowers, but I was no longer able to tell her that dad had sent them, as I did not think she was aware of his death. Somehow, he always managed to jog my memory when I forgot and I would hurry round to the florist!  She would always say how lovely they were.

In the care home, mum wrote some silent notes to a care assistant:

"Dear Sherry, My thoughts again! Time to go home, but where is it? And what is it????I know not!!? One day I will hopefully.  No offence meant – you are lovely people here and thank you for looking after me! And others. You are all so understanding!! And I have a second HOME!!We are lucky *people to be here. From Elsie W. Sincerely yours!!!*

To Sherry at the care home: *Thank you for your interest!! Elsie W.*

*" Jane has gone for a holiday".* (So far from the truth!)

(Once we took Nellie Dean on a holiday with us. Unfortunately, when we reached the holiday let, the beds were made with black sheets. Mum had always liked white linen on her beds and she said: "I'm not sleeping in that! It's like getting into a coffin!"  I had to buy new white sheets before she would sleep in the bed!! I DID SEE HER POINT! At her great age you cannot be too careful!)

And a letter to me that I didn't see:

*Dear Jane, (from Mum in Cornwall). Why couldn't I come home to Surrey with you? I could see*

Sal about somewhere to stay until we find something for me and in any case there is a home nearby I might qualify for! Just a thought!! Cornwall is not a friendly place!! I want so much to be in Surrey. It's really home for me!! Well, I suppose I can go on dreaming. What a life!! I do appreciate your visits. I do know what it's like when your life is so full and you must not neglect your husband!! How I long to be in Surrey again and I think all of the true friends I have made over the years and don't see any more. I don't like Cornwall any more. I suppose it is because I will never be able to go to more places with this dementia and physical uselessness!! Still, perhaps I won't live too much longer. I am in my eighties now so I suppose I've done my stint in life!!

*Luv U! Bye, Mum."*

Note to self :

*"Review my medications. My nurse has moved on. I need to move back to Surrey. I certainly don't need a nursemaid any more - she's made a job of slowing me down. I object to being drugged to sleep or for anything else. Review my medication - Back to Surrey. Emergency. See proper doctor this left to me."*

(Mum was never given any sleeping pills in the care-home)

THE MYSTERY

An old friend, a lady in Australia, would often write letters to mum. Unfortunately, the lady also had Alzheimer's and neither could remember where they had met! Mum could not say who this lady was, only that she knew her from the past. Well, I am up for a good mystery and one day, when I had written to the lady, on behalf of mum, we received a letter back from the lady's son who was enquiring where they had met. It got me thinking and I looked on the internet for the old General Electric Company where Mum worked during the war. I asked my uncle, who also worked at the GEC, and he had some answers. He recognised the name of the lady now living in Australia.

He revealed that Mum and the lady had both worked at the GEC together and he found some pictures. I send the pictures to Australia and the mystery was solved.

I continued to send letters and cards to mum's colleague until, sadly, one day I received a copy of her funeral arrangements. I could not tell Nellie Dean that her old friend had passed away. However, I learned a great deal about the fascinating history of the GEC through this mystery.

Mum's job was checking metals used to make bombs during the war and she hated the work, saying she did not want to help making bombs that kill people.

Nellie Dean's thoughts were becoming jumbled and depression crept in each time I left her. She always saw beauty around her in her life and that alone was perhaps her saving grace.

Nellie Dean wrote: *"His foot was caught in a trap to fear. Who put it there? I know not who, but felt so cross to share care. 'Cause I know not what to do. As I worried in my mind."*

Another letter, written to my brother in Norway, but never sent:

*"This memory thing is very sad and frightening really but I am trying to cope. I have nothing to*

offer you but some money, no real home, like a house, but for what it's worth I shall always love you dearly."

# Chapter 15

## *GAINS AND LOSSES*

The gift of giving.

Nellie Dean was always trying to give me money. Of course I couldn't take it even though she would say she had nothing. Nothing left in life and nothing to give anyone anymore.

I once bought a bunch of flowers for her to give to another lady we knew from the memory cafe. Mum was overjoyed just being able to give something to another person!

From the care home we continued to socialise. The garden club; the art group; memory cafes and other events. Drives in the car and singing in other care homes. We were busy people and needed to be together.

I had finally managed to convince her that she needed to use her walking stick.

She then took it everywhere and it was special to her. Once in a shop in St Austell – an hour's drive away - she hooked her stick onto the counter and we arrived home to find it was lost. I phoned the shop and headed straight back to collect it. It saved me hours of "*Where is my stick*" and was well worth the trip!

Nellie Dean felt the need to walk every day. It seemed to me that it was a reaction to her fear of dementia and she couldn't stay still. It was as if she needed to run away. Nellie Dean walked miles around the care home corridors, declining the offer of a chair. I would be told in no uncertain terms that she *always* did her exercises in the morning, before getting out of bed, and could still touch her toes at 90! She was unstoppable! Nellie Dean only ever did what Nellie Dean wanted to do but she knew exercise was good for her.

One day when I walked with her, I tied her shoe, and she said: *"Thank you! My daughter usually does that for me!"* Conversations became difficult for Nellie Dean. She had lost the ability to follow a story and assumed people were not talking to her because she could no longer remember the gist if the conversations.

One afternoon we went out with an old visiting friend of mums called Penny. We went to The Masons Arms Public House and had a nice walk together in Enfield Park. 10 mins later Mum remembered nothing of it. Said she felt she had been asleep and then just woken up. Cried in the car for not being able to remember. She still felt she had a nice time though. I felt both happy and sad for her. Later in evening I felt depressed and cried, feeling frightened for her future and unable to help her. I desperately wanted things the way they were before dementia struck.

Despite all her efforts to keep fit, mum took a fall while out walking on a footpath. She did not try to save herself – probably a good thing as she fell flat and only had a small cut to her face. It lead me to think about how the brain can alter responses and affect everything we do. It was a great loss to her confidence. The fear of her fall lasted 6 months in her mind and she was convinced she would fall again. Eventually that memory became erased as well. Whilst Nellie Dean could no longer remember family names and occasions, the emotional side of her brain felt fear and protected her for a while from further falls. Many times during that 6 months, Nellie Dean would imagine she was falling again and her walking was shaky. She conceded to having a walker, but eventually recovered enough to dance again.

Nellie Dean would continue to deny any toothache or other pain, when confronted by an appointment with dentist or doctors.

Nellie Dean was left to bear her tooth pain and, after a few months, the offending rotten teeth fell out. She was determined not to have them taken out. Perhaps Nellie Dean remembered the tooth fairy and wanted to keep them under her pillow!! The crisis was all over – till the next time! A similar problem happened with a doctor's appointment for pain too, but was never resolved.

It may take people with memory loss several months to absorb events and facts and fear can step in when no longer able to understand what is happening to them.

FOOD

I continued to cook meals for mum. There were never enough potatoes. I cooked twice as many and there were never any over. Somewhere far back in my family line one of our relatives was Irish so I guess that explains it!

For Nellie Dean, red plates which were suggested to help her eat, would not have helped, as she hated the colour red all her life and its connotations with sleazy women. She would never have any red clothing at all.

Suddenly Nellie Dean disliked Lasagne – previously, one of her favourite foods. Jam tarts were in and Lasagne was a definite out! Chicken soup always remained favourite – perhaps because it was her mother's remedy for all ills. In every meal she ate she discovered *"The black bits"*. Anything with herbs, or a small burnt piece of onion, was not to be eaten. The "black bits" were placed very carefully, all through the meal, on the side of the plate, like foreign objects. I am sure she thought that both I and the care-home cook were trying to poison her! My cooking changed to suit with no herbs or other "poison" in the recipes!! I had to take care not to give her the only white dinner plate with a black speck permanently in the china or it was mayhem!

As time went on, Nellie Dean said she was never hungry – especially if food was served that she didn't want to eat. I discovered a trick of turning her plate around half way through the meal and she continued to eat. Nellie Dean had forgotten family names.

If you think about looking at an illusion of a pattern where, although static, our brains see movement, this is how we all fill in the gaps when we can't take in all the information we are presented with. This is what happens in dementia when connections are broken and gaps will be filled in – sometimes in an appropriate way and sometimes not.

# THE DAMMIT DOLL

Mum had long since been sent a copy of a pattern by her sister Margaret to make a "dammit doll". The dolly was useful at times!

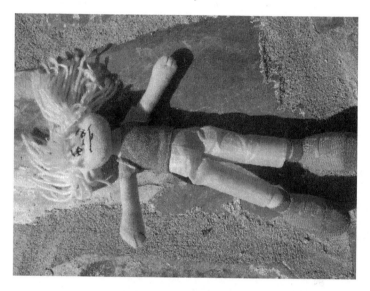

WHEN YOU THINK YOU WANT TO CLIMB THE WALL

OR STAND UP AND SHOUT,

HERE'S A LITTLE 'DAMMIT DOLL' YOU CANNOT DO WITHOUT.

JUST GRASP IT FIRMLY BY THE LEGS AND FIND A PLACE TO 'SLAM IT'

THEN WHACK IT UP AGAINST A WALL SHOUTING

'DAMMIT – DAMMIT - DAMMIT'

F-A-R-T-S

Walking ones were the best! Some days mum would know, but as Nellie Dean, she just let rip! Mum always was a proper lady but Nellie Dean did her best to ignore that!

Like the word Alzheimer's, the word "farts", was something my ladylike mum didn't discuss! As time wore on, she became used to them and even told me a poem about them:

 A little puff of wind, coming from the heart, travels down the backbone and is often called a "f.......t"!

She finally dropped all etiquette and laughed till she "blew off" again!! It has since come to light that someone believes wind can alleviate the symptoms of dementia! Perhaps it has more to do with a good belly laugh!

After mum passed on, I gave away the "half a table" that my father had brought home to her years ago. "Well" she said to him, "What do I want with half a table? What good is that?" She absolutely hated that table, but kept it until the end of her days. I feared it was destined to become mine! With no space for it, I wasn't sure what to do! I revisited mum's care home for a singalong one day and they had an identical table in the entrance for visitors to use when signing in. It was a poor sister to mum's half a table and had seen better days! Although mum hated that half a table, she had looked after it and kept it dusted for years, I saw my chance! "Would you like a "new" half a table for the hall?" I asked the manageress. That half a table was in the boot of my car faster than you could say "free furniture" and I know mum would have been proud that I had finally found a good home for it!

For many years, mum had owned a much-loved coloured dolly, but I don't know where she came from. I christened her Nellie Dean and she went to a good home with one of our ambassador's friends, a lonely lady who would cherish it as mum had. (Thanks Anita!)

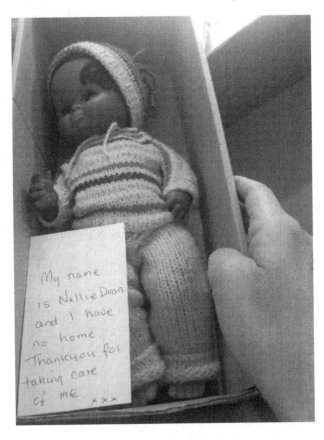

## A long time ago

I thought I knew life and what it held for me. What I didn't know was that there was another plan for me despite what I felt I was destined for! Now in my later years, surprises lurk around every corner. For years my mother looked after me, cared for me and loved me. Then it was my turn as she became more forgetful and her life became confused with dementia. My life has taken on a course not of my making. There are days when I wish I had never heard the word dementia, but still there are things that inspire me and lift my expectations of human nature; make me smile; and gave me a new perspective on my mother's different personalities. I became her memory, the thinker; the doer and I felt the honour. I have met many people since the start of the Purple Angel dementia awareness campaign and have seen how much perseverance, enthusiasm, wit and courage people diagnosed with dementia have. Despite all the difficult times, I remember mostly the joyful days. People with dementia can teach us all so much. To get to know my mother, better than most daughters ever could, and to help her to maintain a dignified life, was a wonderful privilege. On the way I learnt about empathy and patience although I have to say it took me a while! To really know and understand another I believe eludes all of us until we meet adversity. Remembering names and places doesn't matter anymore. They are small fry! What does matter is that we find unconditional love and acceptance of the things which are said, or done, that don't fit in with our own expectations or perception. I learnt to accept the differences dementia had made to my mother.

She had changed but, I too, had also done so.

2016 – My mother was now 95.

May 9th: End of Life Care they said.

May 21st: Eating nothing, taking no fluid at all

May 15th: She said "They're waiting for me"

May 22nd:  A small drink of tea lifted our spirits.

Then, it seemed, nothing.

No Walking, talking, eating, drinking only listening left now.

These were the saddest days, but propped up by all the good times we had shared which I would have missed, were it not for dementia. The good times outweighed the bad.

There was so much I still wanted to say to mum and never seemed to find the right time.

Now I had all the time in the world. I sat by her bed, made sure she was comfortable and played her favourite Nellie Dean on my mobile.

A few days before she died she was murmuring. I heard 2 notes of Nellie Dean and said to her: "That's Nellie Dean you're singing!" Without opening her eyes, she smiled a big gummy smile and I knew she could still hear me.

I told her that I would make sure she was looked after and had no pain. She then said: *"Thank you".* She hadn't spoken for weeks. I told her she did not need to thank me because I loved her. *"I love you too"* she replied. It was the best gift I will ever receive.

Hearing is one of the last things to go and feelings remain till the end of time.

We no longer had anything more we needed to say to each other but, after her funeral, I discovered many notes hidden in her drawings. They were notes saying thank you to the staff that had cared for her and to me, the names of her three children and her thoughts about what was happening to her.

1st June, 2016 the angels took her.

My dear mum, my Nellie Dean, was gone. I was left to ponder all the memories she had left with me.

I look at her paintings on my walls and re-live great days together. The bad times are all gone. One day, maybe, it will happen that I will follow in her footsteps, but I know now, that the things I cherish, will all be lost to me, except one

# -Love-

A poem from my friend:

## A DEEP BREATH IN

(To All Carers/Caregivers around the world)

A deep breath in, a deep breath out
Sometimes that's what it's all about,
To care for someone every day,
Needs so much strength of that I pray,
Carers, Caregivers around the world,
Living daily, on nerves unfurled,
Never knowing what the next hour brings,
What lies ahead, the battle, the stings,
Yet there you are, always there,
To nurse, and comfort, always care,
For people like me who ask too much,
Always needing that loving Crutch,
So from me to you, from deep within,
So sorry for getting under your skin,
It's my illness and not the real me,
I`m still here inside, not the one that you see,
So please forgive and always know,
I will be forever in your debt, my life I owe,
For your kindness, right from the start,
I love you with every piece of my heart,
And to all of you, who work like this,
Please accept my biggest kiss.

©Norrms (Diagnosed with dementia 2007)

Made in the USA
Lexington, KY
30 April 2018